HOW TO GET PREGNANT FAST

Written By: Sam Hall

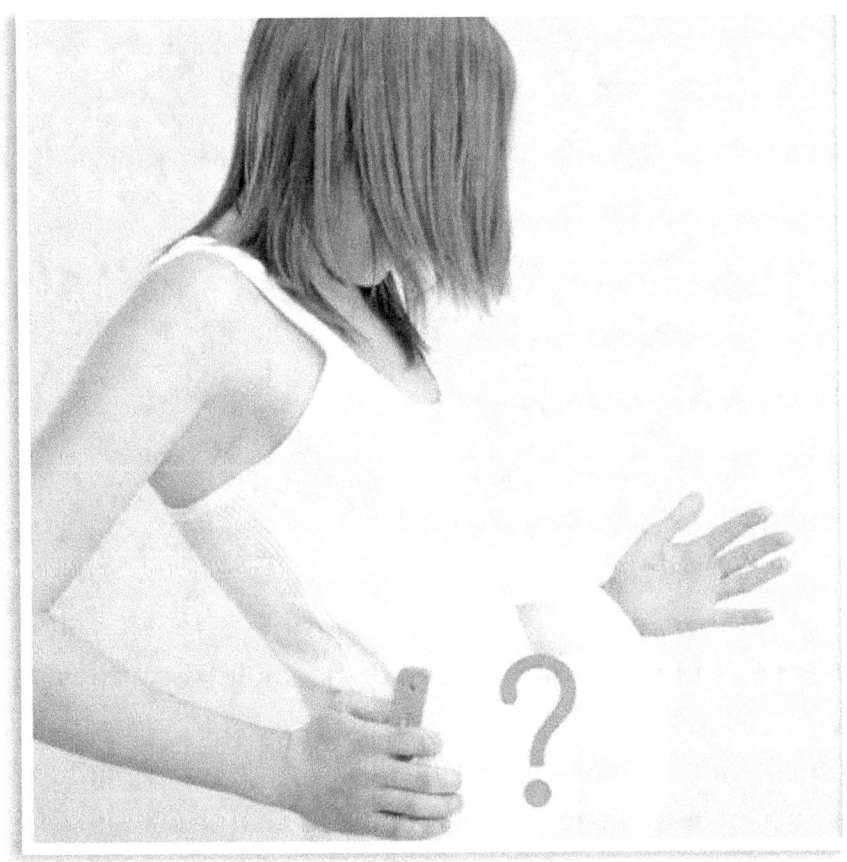

It may seem counterintuitive to the seventeen year old version of yourself, but after years (and perhaps decades) of successfully warding off unwanted pregnancy, you are now ready to bring a little one into the world. The problem is, you're an expert in not having a baby. Plus, you're ready for it to happen right now. So, how do you get started?

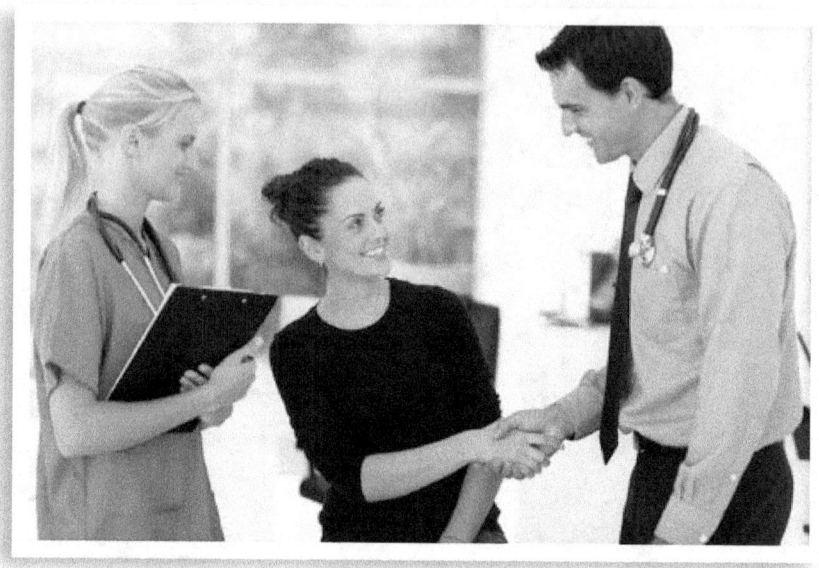

The first bit of advice that any responsible resource will offer you (and I consider myself responsible), is to consult your obstetrician. If you have been on any sort of birth control for a long period of time, you are going to want to learn as much as you can about how to deal with side effects from discontinuing your method. Never stop using a medication without consulting your physician.

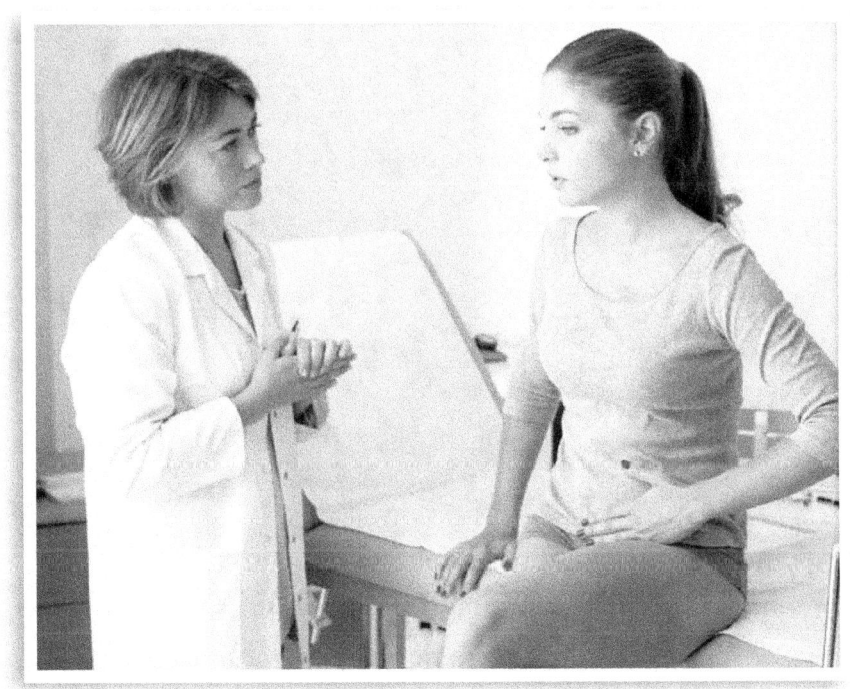

There's another reason for a visit to your gyno: they know your history, and will be able to give you personalized advice on how to move forward. If there are any concerns, it is better to know how to address them at the outset. After all, knowledge is power.

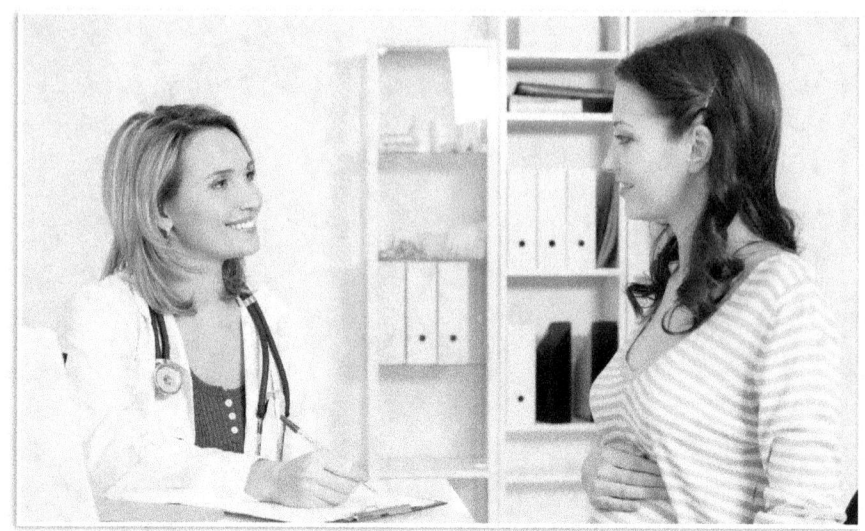

Now that you've scheduled your appointment, let's get down to brass tacks: you need to know how everything works down there. It's been a long time since most of us were in a biology class, and the embarrassment of those first "How Girls' Bodies Work" lessons is probably clouding your memory quite a bit. Even if you think you know all there is to know, take 15 minutes out of your day and google the female reproductive system. I promise, you'll learn something.

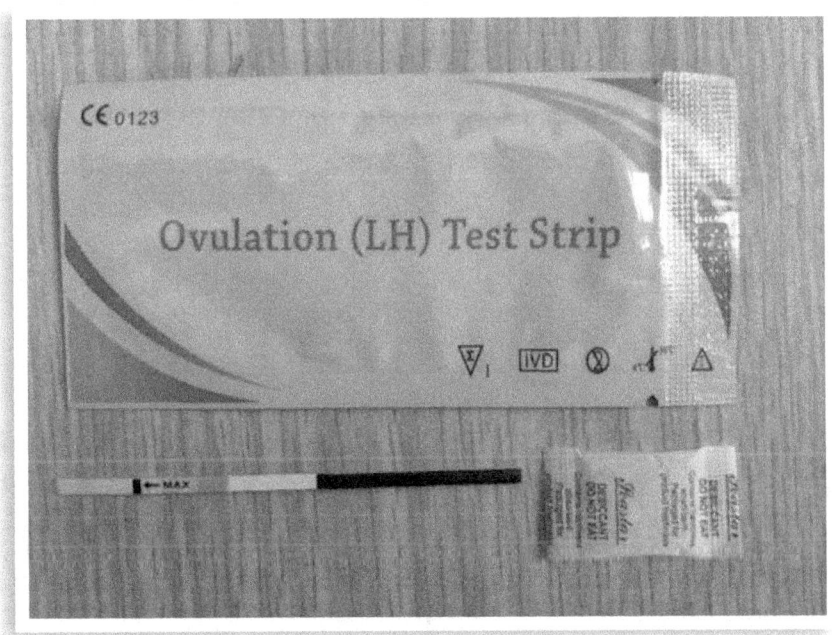

Timing your cycle is the next step to successful pregnancy. This one can be tricky if you're one of us lucky ladies whose bodies eschew any sort of regular rhythm, so keep track for a few months. Generally, you are most fertile during 3 days around the 14th day since your last period. You can buy ovulation tests to track this more closely now. Get it on as often as possible during this period of time especially (though don't make it a chore, and have lots of practice sessions in between to keep things fun).

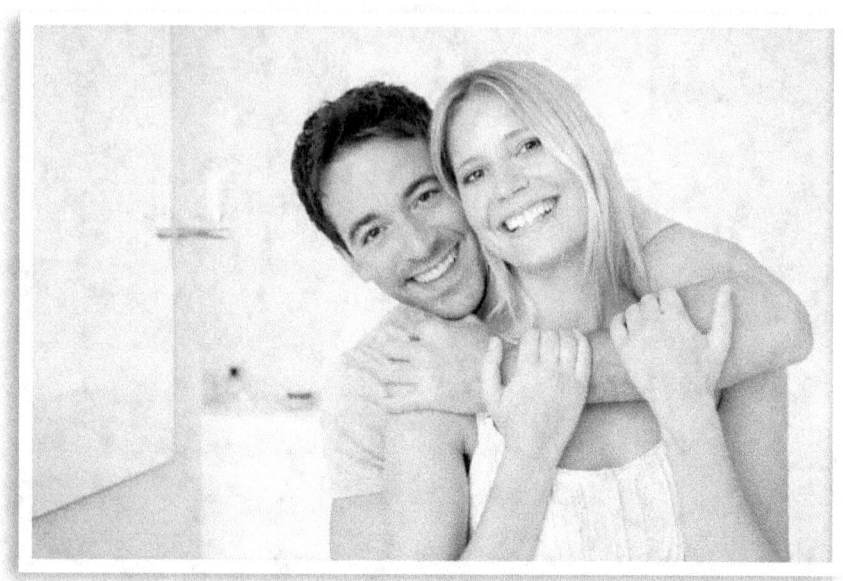

Give yourself a break. Stressing about not getting pregnant right away can have a negative impact on your cycle. No pressure or anything. We all want what we want, especially when it comes to starting our family, but nature has its own rhythm. Each cycle only presents you with a one in five chance of conception, so it takes a while for most people.

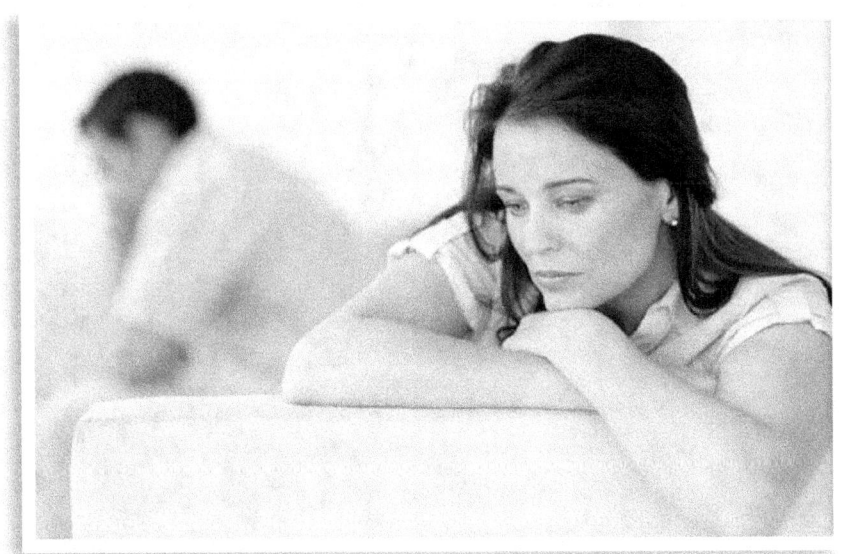

Since it tends to take a long time for the stars to align and a little munchkin to implant itself in your uterus, don't go calling your gynecologist every month demanding answers on how to make it happen. The general rule is to discuss this during your yearly exam. If you're over 35, schedule an appointment every six months while you are trying if you feel the need. Otherwise, live your life and let nature take its course.

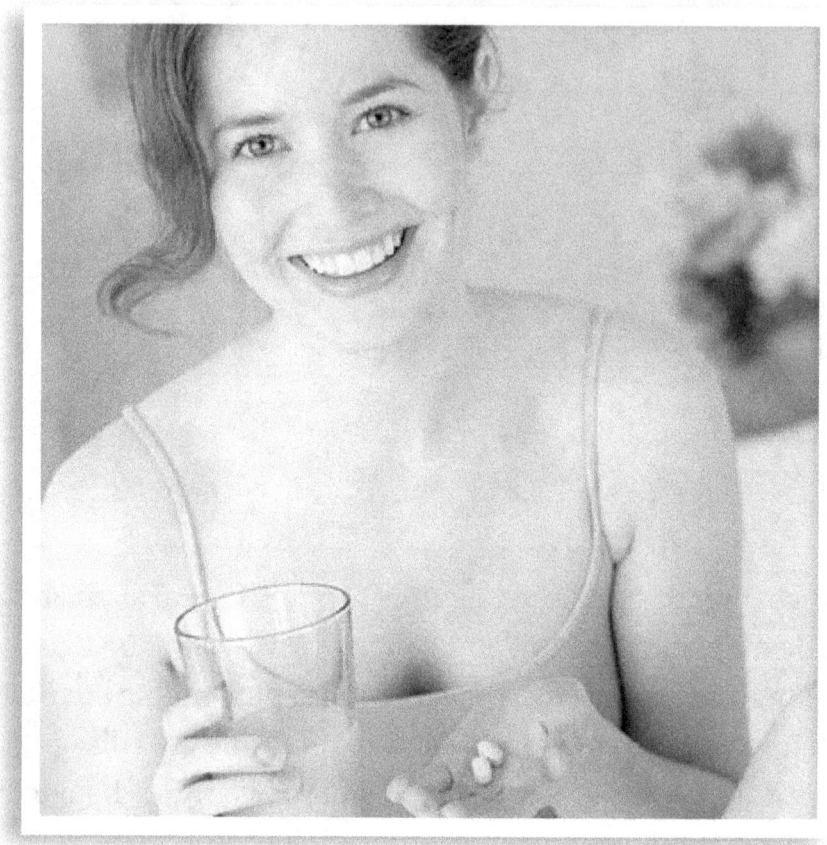

One word: vitamins. Even if you are planning to become pregnant, the first signs often don't show themselves until the 5th or 6th week. These weeks are when the little munchkin's placenta is forming, and the more nutrients you have available to you and your uterus the better off you will be. Your body knows when it is ready to get pregnant, so send it some signs in the form of a daily vitamin ritual.

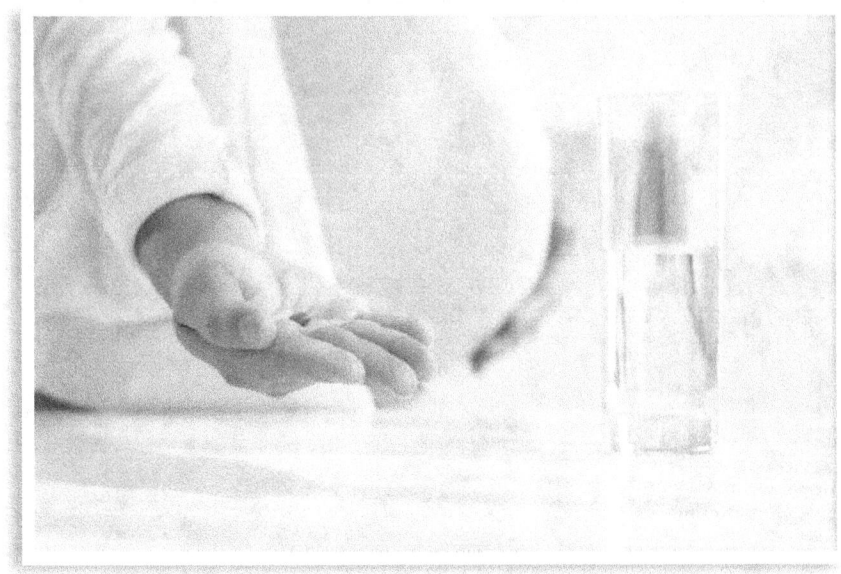

Many women elect to take a prenatal vitamin during this time. My advice is to be careful: prenatal vitamins are more potent than daily multivitamins, and therefore more likely to unsettle your stomach. Find a time of day that works for you (mine is after dinner, but a few hours before bed) when the vitamins don't affect you as severely.

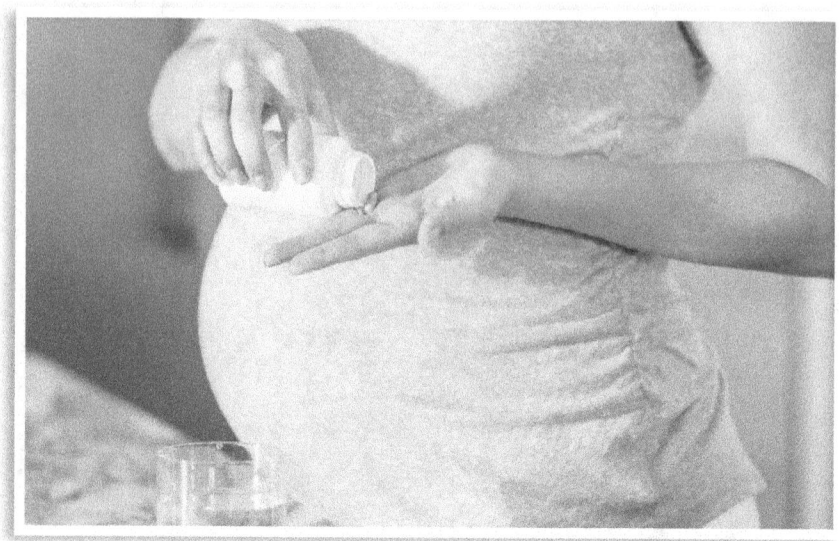

If you elect to continue with your multivitamin for now, consider a folic acid supplement as well. Make sure that you are not overdoing it. Folic acid is proven to reduce the risk of cardiovascular disease in newborn babes.

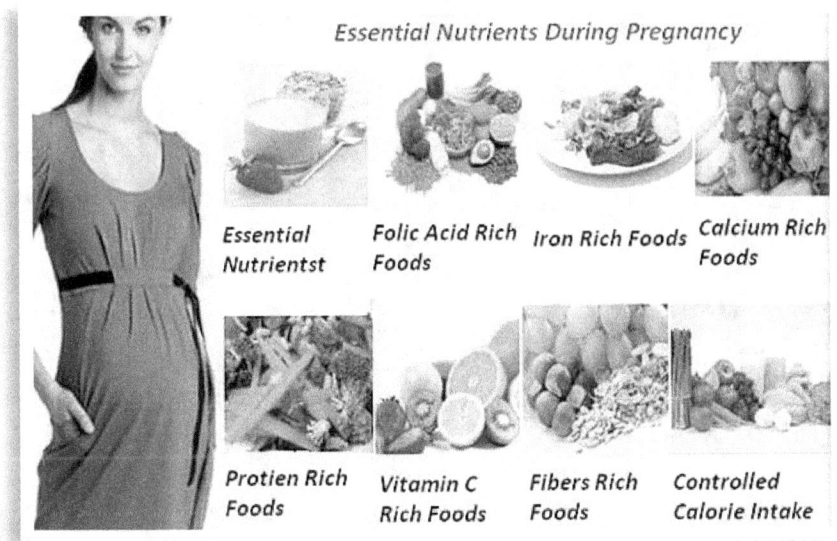

Essential Nutrients During Pregnancy

Essential Nutrientst

Folic Acid Rich Foods

Iron Rich Foods

Calcium Rich Foods

Protien Rich Foods

Vitamin C Rich Foods

Fibers Rich Foods

Controlled Calorie Intake

Examine your diet. An unhealthy body will have a really hard time making another human, so pay attention to what you put into your mouth. There are millions of tips and tricks for types of foods to cause conception, but the bottom line is that you should make sure you are getting the recommended fruits and vegetables, watching your meat and carbohydrate intake, and limiting your sweets. Think of it as practice for dealing with the cravings you'll soon be feeling on a regular basis.

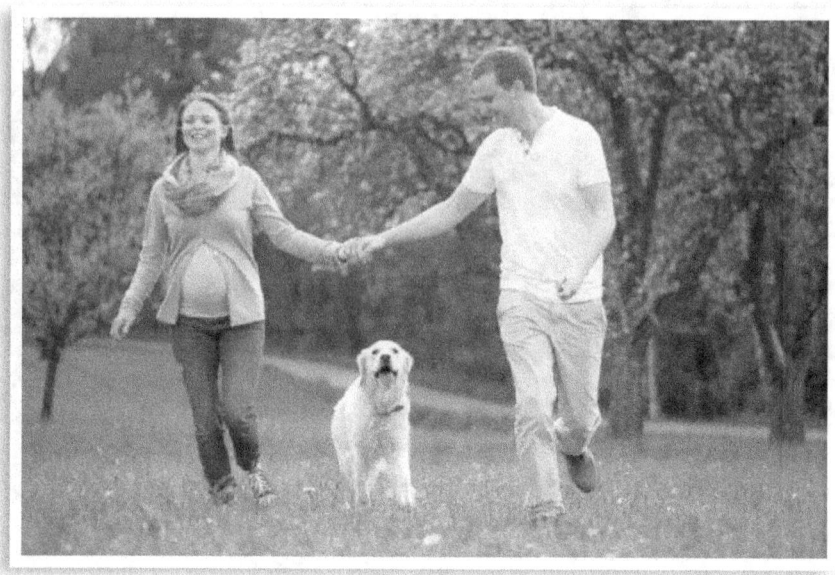

Get moderate exercise. This is probably not the time to start off your kickboxing career, but it is the time to get your cardiovascular system in good order and reduce stress through physical activity. Find an activity that you enjoy and that will help out your body. Bonus points if you and your partner can enjoy this together, and double points if it's something like swimming or walking that you can continue throughout pregnancy.

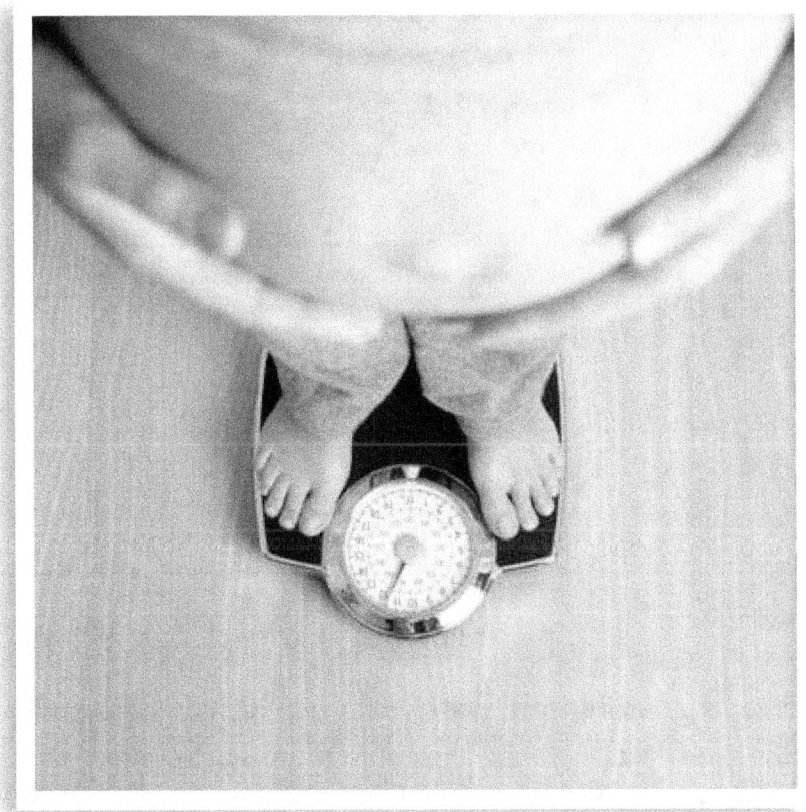

Watch your weight. As though there isn't enough pressure on women to examine the numbers on a scale, now it is actually very important. Talk to your doctor about your ideal weight for conception. If you are underweight, seek advice on how to add pounds in a healthy way (they usually don't advise daily ice cream, though you could get lucky). If you are overweight, see above and make sure to not overdo. After all, stress can make it hard to get healthy as well as pregnant.

Pre-Pregnancy BMI	BMI* (kg/m2) (WHO)	Total Weight Gain Range (lbs)	Rates of Weight Gain* 2nd and 3rd Trimester (Mean Range in lbs/wk)
Underweight	< 18.5	28–40	1 (1–13)
Normal Weight	18.5–24.9	25–35	1 (0.8–1)
Overweight	25.0–29.9	15–25	0.6 (0.4–0.5)
Obese (includes all classes	> 30.0	11–20	0.5 (0.4–0.5)

'*Women with a BMI of 40 or more should gain no more than 10-15 pounds

There is a good reason to strive for a healthy weight. Studies have shown that women with a BMI higher than 35 can take twice as long to conceive, while a woman with a BMI lower than 19 can take four times as long. Women who are overweight tend to produce more estrogen which can interfere with fertility, while underweight women often experience unreliable ovulation cycles.

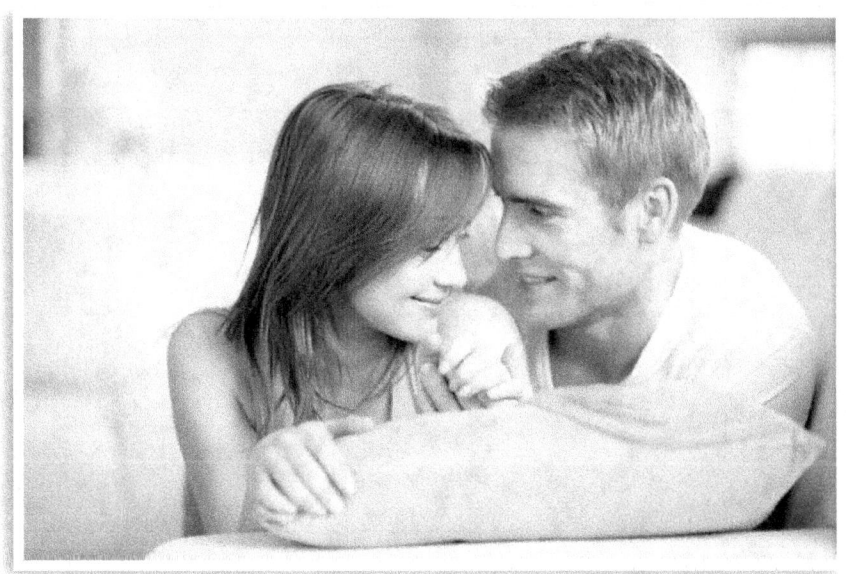

Master your timing. Many modern authorities now suggest that more successful couples have sex every other day during the fertile window (four or five days prior to ovulation). The percentage of successful pregnancies differs by about 4%, so this isn't necessarily a hard and fast rule. However, it could give you an edge if you've been trying for a while.

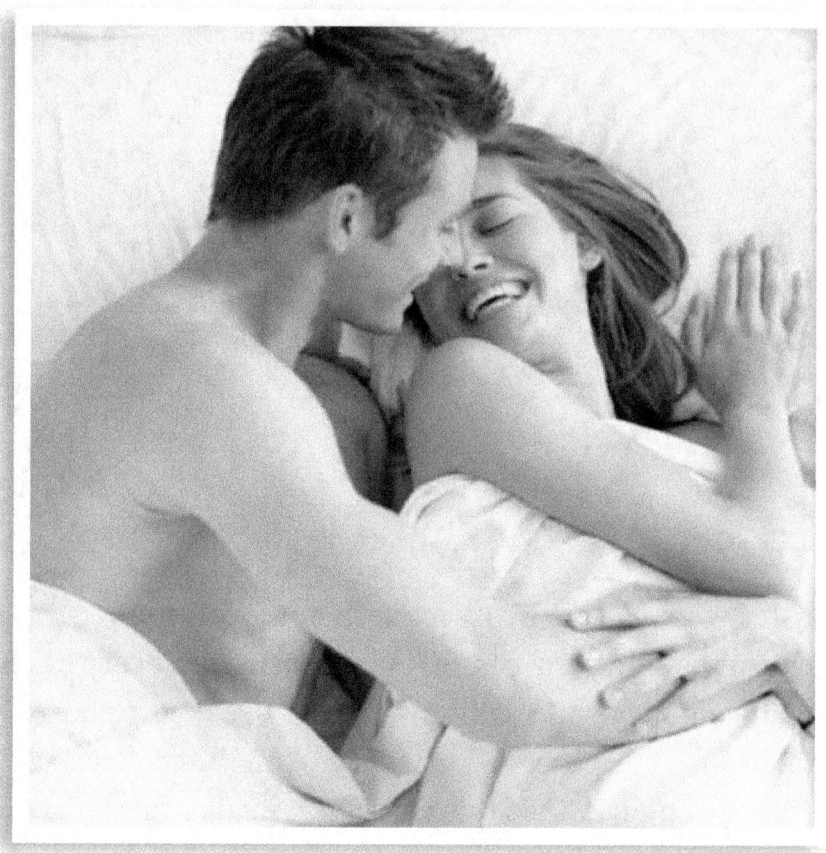

Don't forget the romance. There is nothing less sexy than when making love becomes a chore. It's hard to avoid this when you're scheduling your sessions to a calendar. However, you will enjoy the experience of babymaking more if you can tap into the passion that brought you two together in the first place. After all, that passion is the foundation for the family that you are creating together.

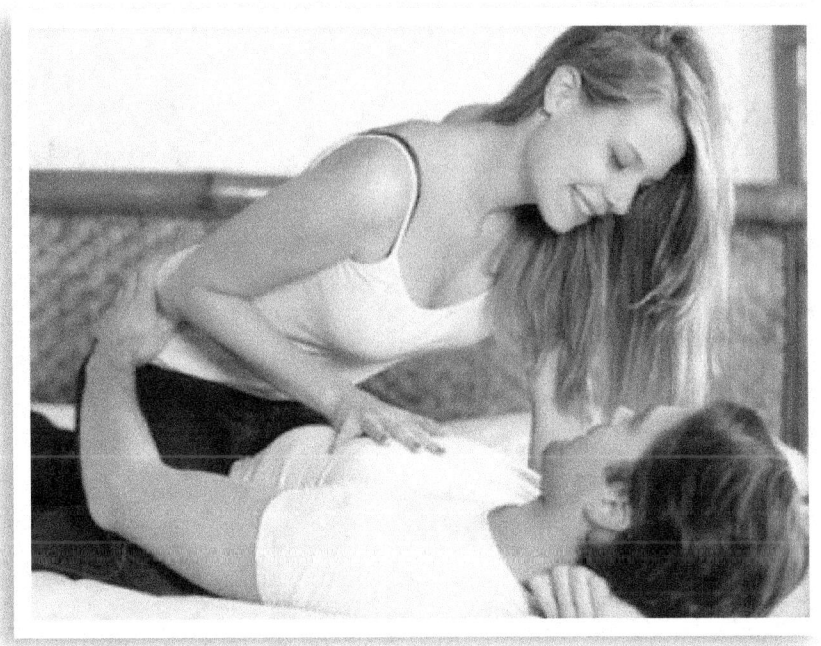

Make your sex count. The pulsing motions that are fired off during your orgasm power the little sperm onto their destination, so make sure you're getting your fill with each sex act. Additionally, pay attention to your lubricant: most are a barrier to the little swimmers, even if they don't contain spermicide. If lube is a necessity, find one that is sperm friendly. Alternatively, put in a little extra time at the outset so that you don't need any assistance.

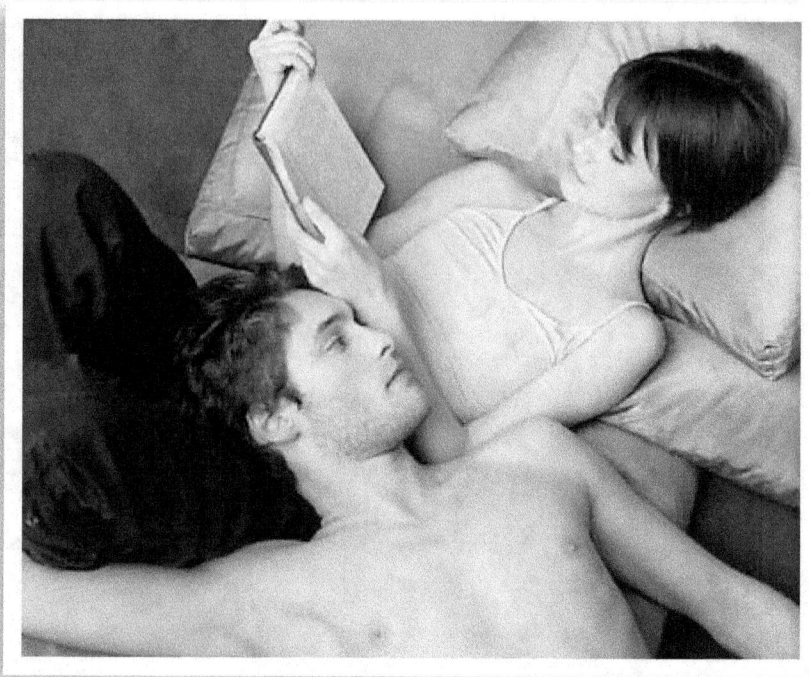

Rest and relax afterwards. Instead of popping up out of bed and moving on with your day, take advantage of the opportunity to lay back with your pelvis propped up on a pillow. Grab a book and let gravity help those baby making minions reach their destination.

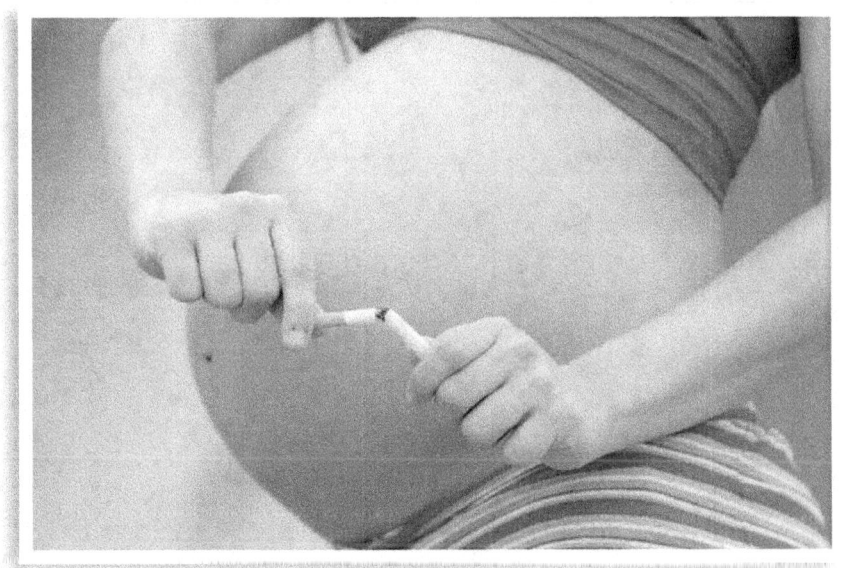

Stop smoking. After all, you are preparing to bring a baby into the world, and pregnant women are greatly discouraged from this unhealthy habit. Aside from that, there have been studies that show that smoking can speed up egg loss in women of childbearing years. Your heart, lungs, and future baby will all thank you.

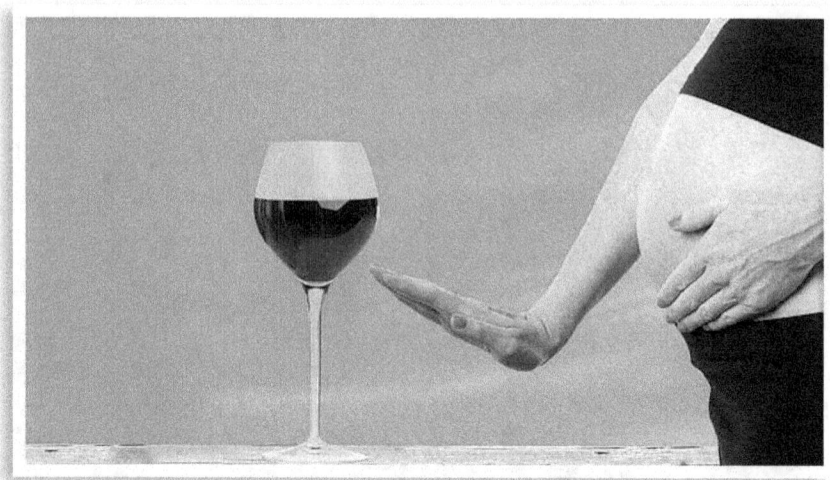

Stop drinking alcohol. There are several authorities that state that even moderate drinking can reduce a woman's risk of conception. Think of it as practice, as there is no amount of alcohol that is generally considered safe during pregnancy anyway, and you'll have to curb your consumption of sweet sweet booze during breastfeeding.

Thank You!

We hope you enjoyed the book! All pictures and words were lovingly put together by experts who really love what they do! We really hope you learned something new today!

We would really appreciate it, if you could PLEASE take the time to let us know how we're doing by leaving a review on the Amazon website. We appreciate any comments you may have – what you enjoyed about the book, what additions you would have liked to have seen and what you would like to see in future publications.

Any comments will help understand better what you and your kids most enjoy and allows us to better provide exactly what you want!

Thought Junction Publishing

A NOTE FROM THE WRITER

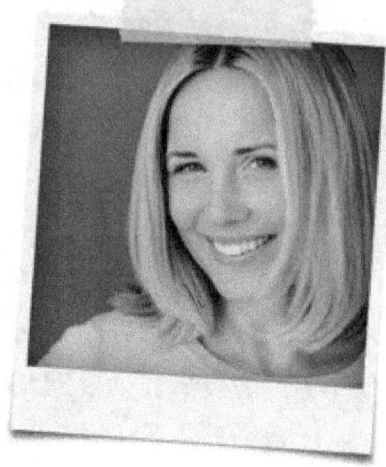

Sam's life revolves around her family, devoted mother of 3 - Noah (6), Oscar (3) and Poppy (11months) - she writes in a real way, aiming to answer the questions that other books don't cover, to fill in the blanks and inform parents and parents-to-be of the truth about raising children in the modern world.

Sam's writings emphasize that the readers are not alone - that there is a community of support available, and other people to talk to who can help, support and assist.

When she's not writing books, Sam is an advisor and avid blogger for Ideal Parent - http://ideal-parent.com - spreading support, care and advice across the web!

Join Sam on Ideal Parent and keep an eye out for her books - she's on a mission to help parents worldwide - join her and spread the word!

www.ingramcontent.com/pod-product-compliance
Lightning Source LLC
Chambersburg PA
CBHW061954280526
45787CB00004B/1860